A Survivor's

Journey of Hope

Winning the Battle of Cancer one Cure at a Time!

****

Shanda L. Wright

Winner *** Miracle *** Victorious One

A Survivor's, Journey of Hope

Winning the Battle of Cancer one Cure at a Time

ISBN-13:978-1548447373

Printed in the United States (U.S.)

Winning the Battle of Cancer one Cure at a Time!

My journey with cancer taught me many positive things. Things I thought I already knew but never put fully into practice as I do today. Cancer tends to put things in perspective. It's been an enormous learning curve. A journey I had to go through that changed my life. Having cancer changed everything for me: My attitude, my pride, and I realized sitting at home and crying was not going to solve anything so I had to focus on winning the battle.

I WON!

I SURVIVED!

I AM VICTORIOUS!

Inspirational Prayer

Lord of all power, so many people are hurt with aching pain, and their bodies aren't functioning as it should due to their breast cancer diagnosis. Heal them, mend their heart, bodies, and minds. Lord, grant them days of better health and renewed strength. Dear God, give them extra measures of patience, endurance, and perseverance. When their energy levels are low, please pour your power into them to uplift the heavy burdens on their hearts. Shine through me that every person I meet may feel your presence in my soul. Guide every doctor's decision, response, effort, and any discussion which I have with them before your Glory. In Jesus name AMEN!

Table of Contents

Dedication

Introduction

Chapters

Dedication

This book is dedicated to all cancer survivors and in honor of loved ones as well as families who lost a loved one in their battle to fight back against cancer. A Survivor's Journey of Hope was written to ensure that a journey of hope never ends because it's good when other survivors can share their stories of wisdom, hope, and healing as a means of knowing how to survive through the process. One has to travel down the pathways in order to be able to encourage others whom may feel a burning oil deep down inside to make ultimate decisions of the countless hours when going through weeks of treatments. There will be some bumps in the road that will slow down the progress along the Journey, but having a positive mindset and support from others makes the process flow easier. For those whom take the time to

read this book and are going through this walk of

healing, I pray it helps build the strength, courage,

and hope to become a fearless faith fighter along the

"Journey of Hope".

INTRODUCTION

My life changed after hearing the devastating news, "You Have Cancer!" It seemed like a dream but after crying for three long days, I had to face reality and realized that even strong warriors have to face battles too. My motto H.O.P.E. is Helping Other People Embrace. My story is helping Women and Men of Strength & Grace to Inspire Others to Live Healthy Lives. My survivorship has made me become a Fearless Faith Fighter. After viewers read this book "A Survivor's Journey of Hope", it is a means to help them gain strength to endure there process and know that in the midst of their battle there's still hope. A means to know that not every illness is a deathful situation but there are brighter days ahead but one must fight to become a winner over any situation.

Chapter 1

Survivor's Story: A Living Testimony

At the age of 41 years old, on July 23, 2009, I was diagnosed with stage II breast cancer. When I first heard the words, "You Have Breast Cancer", I cried hysterically! I had become a ball of emotions because I was so afraid; afraid of death! This was a very stressful moment but I, Shanda L. Wright had to gain a sense of strength. I had to run to my source of strength (God). I trusted God's word **Matthew 17:20**, "Ye have faith as a grain of a mustard seed." However, I knew that overcoming this battle with cancer was not going to be easy, but I had faith that it was possible! On August 17, 2009, I had my first surgery which was a lumpectomy to remove the tumor, lymph nodes, and a double mastectomy where

I chose to have both breasts removed due to a 20% chance of recurrence. I was in so much pain, I couldn't even lay down to rest without taking medication from this surgery which took approximately six weeks to heal. After which, I had to wear prosthesis for months before I started my reconstruction but it was my Faith that got me through.

Coping with chemotherapy from September 17, 2009-January 21, 2010 for four months, every fourteen days, for four hours per day made my body suffer from fatigue, nausea & lack of appetite. After my first treatment was completed, I lost all of my hair and I started to feel a bit insecure! After all, this was so new to me! I've always had a head full of hair. I was insecure about what people would think of me when they saw me. After taking weeks of treatments the discoloration of my skin began to change but overtime it changed back. I had to realize that it was not the beauty on the outside that made me look good, but it was all the beauty deep down on the inside, because God made me who I am with a clean pure heart, good spirit, and pleasant personality. However, it took a lot of prayer for me to gain the confidence needed to feel good on the inside. Within that four month period I lost thirty pounds and many days I felt like giving up and throwing in the towel. I've endured many sleepless nights and aching pain in my legs producing the inability for me to walk on some days. There were plenty days that I wanted to give up, but I began to think about Matthew 27, the chapter which discusses the crucifixion of Jesus and all the pain & anguish He faced prior to and during his crucifixion.

Reminiscing on what Jesus had gone through to save his people is what gave me strength to keep pushing.

Coping with radiation from February 15-April 1, 2010, traveling up and down the dangerous highway for seven long weeks, thirty minutes per day on Monday- Friday left my body severely fatigue but I realize that all my weakness was to make me stronger because it says in **John 11:4,** "This sickness is not unto death, but for the glory of God." On June 7, 2011, I had undergone my first reconstruction surgery to have tissue expanders inserted and a latissimus flap procedure underneath the back muscle. During this procedure, my skin tissue was stretched from the skin of my back, to my chest wall. In other words, the doctor pulled skin from my backside and it stretched all the way to the front of my chest. The pain that I felt was indescribable! I was in so much pain from the stitches across my chest and the dissolvable staples across my back, along with weeks of saline solutions pumped by a needle to enlarge my breast to a B cup size. There were many days that I cried, and I have a high tolerance for pain! I had to continue with another surgery on April 17, 2012 which was my second reconstruction surgery to have the tissue expanders removed and silicone implants inserted. The song, "Never Would Have Made It" by renowned gospel artist Marvin Sapp is what kept me going.

On June 11, 2014, I completed my last doctor visit and I celebrated! I can truly say that I am stronger because I chose to live and not die. I am so much wiser because of my knowledge and understanding. I'm healed because of **Isaiah 53:5**, and on March 30, 2017, I completed the final surgery to get my revisions, areola reconstruction, and breast lift which took weeks to heal and followed by other minor procedures & follow-ups visit to complete but I survived.

On July 23, 2017, I celebrated being a survivor of 8 years! I am truly a living testimony and have written this book to inspire and encourage other women like me who have been diagnosed with Breast Cancer. I am here today, alive and well to spread the message of hope to let others know that Breast Cancer is not the end of the world, but the beginning of a new journey of hope!

In 2009, cancer crept into my body but I managed to walk away. And suddenly the weight begins to creep back, hair loss grew back and after a while I looked in the mirror and realized. WOW! After all those hurts, scars, and bruises, after all of those trails, I really made it through, I DID IT! I survived that which was supposed to kill me. So I straightened my crown and walked away like one touch chic.

Chapter 2

Spin Straw into Gold

Spin straw into gold is an emotional recovery state of mindset. Cancer survivor individuals have stories which they can share and inspire others to uplift their spirits from sisterhood to sisterhood. After all my surgeries, chemotherapy treatments, radiation treatments, four step reconstruction process and follow-up visits I was in an emotional state but sharing my own personal experiences and encouraging others with my stories through the community helped me to realize it's okay to shed a few tears. During my cancer journey, I was also going through a divorce process, going back and forth to the doctor taking test after test and all of this had put me in a stressful situation. I thought

I was about to lose my mind. Before I got my biopsy results, I thought I had it all together, but on the day of the phone call I immediately gave my God-sister permission to take the call. When she hung up the phone with my physician's office, she looked at me strangely and said, "Yes it is cancer". I remember falling to my knees just like it was yesterday in the hallway of my workplace crying out to God. At that moment I could care less! I began to cry for three long days but I realized I had to pull myself together because I thought about when Jesus rose on the third day with all power in his hands. I was reminded that God won't put no more on me than I could bare because it says in: **Psalm 30:5, "**For his anger is but for a moment; His favor is for a life-time; weeping may tarry for the night, but joy cometh in the morning." I'm so grateful to have a sister that worked in the medical field and she took the initiative to help me through the process at such a dreadful time in my life. I had to swallow a hard pill because three (3) days before my surgery to have the lymph nodes and tumor removed, my divorce was finalized. This was a very emotional, stressful and discouraging time in my life. The emotional recovery from breast cancer is a big experience to go through but always remember that you have the power to spin straw into gold.

Chapter 3

Early Detection

In early detection, breast cancer is the most common kind of cancer in women. This is just some of the most common information to know regarding breast cancer. Early detection saves lives, it's just that simple. If any diagnosis is caught early, the risk of a five (5) year survival rate is almost 100% being cancer-free. It is extremely important for every woman to know their body and reduce the personal experience risk of getting breast cancer. There are self-exams which every woman can better prepare themselves and take the initiative precautions. A lump is not the only sign to be determined, yet it's a sense of knowing how to feel, see and know how to find it.

Performing monthly breast self-exams is an easy way to easily identify any changes in the breast.

All women should know the symptoms and signs of breast cancer and take the time to further find resources and pamphlets for self-checks. Women should perform a self-breast exam daily, weekly, and monthly. Anytime a woman discovers abnormalities, it's just a matter of taking the time to make an appointment with their primary physician for further testing procedures. A change in the breast, nipple, or underarm area describes similar signs but not all lumps are cancerous. When looking for certain unexplainable changes, it is mostly common in the skin of the breast, areola, or nipple that becomes swollen or reddish around the appearance areas. A woman should never second guess the symptoms but find the time to go get tested by mammogram screenings or even get a bioscopy done to verify if any lumps are cancerous. Getting a medical examination can be very nerve wrecking and stressful but getting an x-ray allows yourself to be confident especially if a qualified specialist examines the breast tissues for any suspicious areas. Regular screening tests, along with follow-up tests and treatment if diagnosed, reduces your chance of suffering from or dying from breast cancer. Some woman don't realize the lack of risk of getting breast cancer is to change their diet because some of the foods which we all eat builds up cancerous cells. A healthy lifestyle decreases the risk of breast cancer and any other illnesses from attacking the body. Daily exercises is one major importance for all men and women to do at least 30-45 minutes per day if possible to prevent such a dreadful illness disease. Breast cancer screening is only recommended for some men at very high risk due to an inherited gene or a strong family history of breast cancer.

Many people in today's society are unaware of the breast cancer symptoms and signs because it can vary from person to person. Some of the signs are as follows:

- **Changes in the skin areas**

- **Swelling in one or both breast**

- **Increase cup breast size of the breast changes overtime from maturity as a teenager to adulthood over periods of time**

- **Discharges in one's nipples other than the norm when a woman is going through pregnancy**

- **Painfulness**

- **Buildup of tissues in the breast**

These are all unaware signs and symptoms to specifically be aware of risk factors which may cause numerous conditions to occur. Early detection has steps and a less chance of finding breast cancer before it spreads. The steps are as follows:

- **Symptoms and Signs**

- **How to perform a breast self-exam**

- **Clinical breast exam**

- **Mammogram**

- **Healthy Balanced Eating Habits**

- **Exercise**

According to the National Breast Cancer Foundation, one out of eight women can be diagnosed with breast cancer in her lifetime. Once women reach the age of 30 plus years, it is highly recommended to get a mammogram. Some women have a higher risk of getting breast cancer than others. Breast cancer is sometimes found after symptoms appear, but many women with breast cancer have no symptoms at all. This is why regular yearly breast cancer screenings is so important.

Taking the time to give self-breast checks can change lives and provide hope and support to those that fight to live and not die. There are other options to find out for sure if one has positive cancerous cells by scheduling a 3D mammography exam which results can be given within less than two weeks so every woman can have a peace of mind. A tissue biopsy is another means of clarity to determine if the required testing is cancerous and further treatments are necessarily needed immediately. After being diagnosed with breast cancer, patients receive a treatment plan to help them beat the disease. Frequently this involves surgery to remove the cancer tumor and a form of breast reconstruction performed by experienced general and plastic surgeons.

Many women face breast cancer with the hope and care they need to make the best decisions to protect their precious lives. Most women who develop breast cancer do not have any known risk factors or a history of the disease in their families. Breast cancer has potentially impacted people close to us. We have mothers, sisters, aunts, cousins, & friends who can possibly be affected by this dreadful disease. Many times whether it's you or a loved one, a newly diagnose of breast cancer involves undergoing treatments and follow-up appointments of the breast cancer recurrence which leads to lots of questions.

Breast cancer is a real disease that affects real people in our communities but there are preventive ways from allowing it to invade the bodies in the near future generations. Many times people who need someone to talk to about their breast cancer diagnosis, finds it difficult to communicate such news with those they can trust and have confidentiality. There are non-profit organizations that supports many people diagnosed with breast cancer and has a potential to impact many lives. For instance, the American Cancer Society has many representatives on duty who are willing to help and be a listening ear during countless hours when there is no friend or family member available at that point in time. Most individuals should know the importance of early detection to decrease the risk of getting breast cancer because there are four different stages (Stage 0-4) and stage 4 being the highest risk but know that it does not affect every individual the same way. The following stages of breast cancer are listed as follows:

Stage 0 Breast Cancer

- Breast cancer stages start at 0 when the abnormal cancerous cells are still within the non-invasive part of the breast.

Stage I Breast Cancer

- When the cancer cells break through and invade other surrounding tissue areas the tumor begins to increase to 2 cm but cancer is still within the boundaries of the breast.

- Stage I contains no lymph node involved and every minute counts because the cancerous cells begins to spread out into other lymph nodes.

Stage II Breast Cancer

- When one is diagnosed with Stage II breast cancer the tumor is 2-5 cm with lymph nodes involved.

- When the tumor is larger than 2 cm without lymph node involvement but not attached to the chest wall, it will cause a breast cancer diagnosis.

- When a tumor is discovered between stages I and II, the chances for a successful treatment is at its highest risk.

Stage III Breast Cancer

- Stage III has a tumor which is less than 5 cm and can spread up to 5-9 lymph nodes.

- Stage III tumor then begins to grow into the chest wall without lymph node involvement.

- Stage III tumors can be any size and spread up to 10 or more lymph nodes in many areas under the underarm.
- At this stage level the cancer cells begin to reach out beyond the breast and some of the lymph nodes begin to become invaded.

Stage IV Breast Cancer

- When cancer reaches this stage, the cancer begins to spread beyond the breast, lymph nodes and other organs of the body that may include the brain, lungs or liver. Some individuals manage to bounce back and live many years and some are not able to survive. What breast cancer can look and feel like during abnormal recognition but don't panic because some changes are normal but never hesitate to show your doctor. A cancerous lump usually feels hard and immovable like the

size of a lemon seed which over time the size
increases from a stage 0 to stage 4.

Symptoms to notice are as follows:

- **Feeling a thick mass**

- **Indentation**

- **Skin Erosion**

- **Redness or Heat**

- **Unexpected fluid or tissues**

- **Dimpling**

- **Bumps**

- **Growing Veins**
- **Retracted Nipple**
- **New shape/size**
- **Peeling of the skin**
- **Hidden lumps**

The list on the previous page are most common
signs of breast cancer and some symptoms can be

seen rather than felt by oneself or a physician. Getting

a mammogram can determine a lump and knowing

yourself and allow the mammograms to determine if

there's any diagnosis. Women should take the time to

do their own research so they can have a peace of

mind and get complete clarity for such a diagnostic

testing. There's no individual that wants to receive

the devastating news, "You have Cancer". It is very

important for all individuals including men and

women to get tested because men can get breast

cancer too. It is okay to ask as many questions

necessary to get a better understanding and know the

difference, options of any or all treatments if needed.

Whether you've never had breast cancer and want to

increase your odds of early detection, you've recently

been diagnosed, or you are in the midst of treatment

and follow-up, you know that breast cancer and

medical tests go hand in hand. Learn how to detect cancer early when it is most treatable. When dealing with cancer risk it can be scary or overwhelming, but believe it or not this information and resources is comforting, empowering, and lifesaving. It is better to be safe than sorry, so be proactive!

Chapter 4

Health and Wellness

Many times one tries to strive and maintain
through the process of survival but making every
moment count to nurture yourself back to health to
have a healthy lifestyle is what's very important.
Every woman, child, or man should get advice to
have a well balance happy life. Health and wellness is
based on great fitness of daily exercise and
maintaining a good nutritious diet. Taking the time to
workout at least four times a week provides a good
means to improve one's overall health and well-
being. There are so many experts and specialists
whom can offer the best options of health and
wellness when facing breast cancer. In many cases,
physicians are so supportive to their patients and they

offer support through recommendations which may also be very helpful. Sometimes attending support groups help sooth a patient's mindset and willingness to share stories of inspiration and informative health and wellness information that will be beneficial to others.

Middle aged women are already at risk for breast cancer, but just being able to embrace and nurture each other is a heathy start to a healthy lifestyle. There are discovery facts on the diagnosis, how it is treated, and how it can be prevented. Getting educated is a healthy plan to get supportive care to complete one's medical treatment, annual health screenings, self-checks and knowing some of the symptoms can help you stay ahead of the breast cancer or catch it early on. Physicians try to do their very best and give the best advice for happy and healthy living for women, men, and children's health. Many times people need to live healthier lives by doing their own research of health tip's and find ways to personally take care of themselves through wellness, fitness and change their diets.

Knowing the importance of health and wellness is like having a good overall connection of one's well-being and health. This takes good understanding of your health, nutrition, physical activity and wellness in your daily life. We must understand how important it is to live a healthy life. The ability to adopt healthy eating and drinking habits (fruits, vegetables, plenty of water, etc.), and exercise for healthiness at least 30-45 minutes per day is extremely important. There is no excuse as cancer does not discriminate, so we must be proactive by adopting good habits to prevent illness.

People, both young and old are getting diagnosed with breast cancer all over the United States. Those are scary statistics to think about because breast cancer has potential to impact people's lives whom are close to us. We have mothers, sisters, aunts, cousins, and friends but believe it or not men can get breast cancer too. Breast cancer is a real disease that affects real people in our community.

Physicals are very important but mammograms are lifesaving screening access to you which your primary physicians will gladly give you a referral. All of the oncologist, chemotherapist and plastic surgeons are very helpful, caring and it makes the treatments and other procedures go much smoother because it gives you a chance to meet other cancer patients.

I remember walking into my radiologist appointment early one morning and the tears would not stop flowing and the secretary allowed me to sit in her office until I stopped crying and she immediately gave me a hug and encouraging words. I begin to start crying once again but I knew I had to fight considering I had to go every morning at 8a.m. This gave me some relief to know that my doctors and his staff cared 100%. This helps a lot to get back to a healthy and wellness state of mindset whether physically and/or emotionally. I pray daily for those that are currently taking treatments because not everyone can handle such illnesses without going through being depressed or just lost for words. Health and wellness services is provided to all cancer patients with the respect of their identity, race, color, creed, religion, national origin, gender identity, sexual orientation, age, disability, citizenship status and socioeconomic status. No one should not be denied to receive services no matter what.

The beginning stage of health and wellness is to live life to the fullest, be healthy and be happy. Don't allow certain diagnosis, diseases or disorders to hinder your lifestyle. In life most struggles are hard but real and life's realness causes troubling thoughts but make the time to get treatments to live a productive life. Some people dread the things which are going on in their personal lives but many times others like me, share their health stories and inspire others to get on track with healthy diets, healthy relationships and learn how to shape up your own personal health.

Chapter 5

Support System

As it relates to the healing process for breast cancer, SUPPORT SYSTEM are two of the most important words for individuals going through an emotional state and needs countless hours of support. Before confiding in someone, it is important to consider the steps in selecting supportive, trustworthy family and friends because there are times an individual begins to have stressful moments and sleepless nights during different hours of the day or night due to the diagnosis. I can't express it enough to make sure the person is trustworthy and supportive because the individual is really going through a tough time in his or her life and that support system must be able to handle any and all odds of emotions from the cancer patient.

The willingness to become a strong support system simply means when things aren't going well or the patient is just not feeling that great and need support and encouragement at that very moment, the supporter will be there to offer encouragement of some sort. This is a position that one must be able and ready to fulfill at any given time. As I recovered from my illness, I offered support to other women who had walked a mile in my shoes. I remember having to turn my back or even just walk out of the room to keep the patient from seeing my tears. I felt this was the best option at that moment. No one really knows what cancer patients go through unless they had to go through it as well. The pain can be excruciating, so ongoing support is needed. Sometimes this can be short or long term support because keeping the patient calm and comfortable at all times is the best healing process.

The importance of having a good support system is pivotal because friendship is the root of a long lasting relationship that provides for a deeper closeness between the two individuals. It deepens both their strength and their friendship to make their strong relationship last forever. Having a good support system simply means that people don't always need advice. Sometimes all they need is a hand to hold, ear to listen and a heart to understand them. Often times a person needs someone to simply be there; not to fix anything, or to do anything in particular but just to let them feel cared for and supported.

A breast cancer diagnosis is the start of an incredibly difficult period for a patient and her family because it affects everyone. One important factor way for a patient to emotionally manage and maintain her diagnosis is to be surrounded by a strong support system. Some patients have family and friends that they can depend on and don't expect anything in return. Having a strong support system helps women feel taken care of during their difficult vulnerable time in their life. Every woman has a different cancer experience and need a different type of support system. Many times all women can think about is all the scars on their bodies and trying to find ways to cope with it all.

The best solution is to share, learn, support and sometimes the best medicine is talking to someone who's been there and can be reliable. These are some emotional supporters to rely on:

- **Survivors**

- **Confidentiality**

- **Caregiver Support**

- **Patient Support**

- **Family Support**

- **Friends of family support**

Support groups can be very helpful and resourceful for others that have been diagnosed with breast cancer. Support groups can provide information and education of what to expect with chemotherapy and health tips on how to cope with treatments. This helps to encourage other people to share their feelings. There should be someone or groups in your surrounding community and be a powerful force for healing but this is not for everyone because some people prefer to have their medical

history private.

Chapter 6

Live, Laugh, Learn & Love

Many survivors and caregivers are drained after weeks and/or months of treatments and just need a place to rest, relax, rejuvenate, and prepare their mindsets to be well taken care of and healed properly. Eventually, survivors and caregivers need a weekend vacation to laugh, live, and love again. As a survivor, I've found myself spending my spare time helping others and their families cope with the devastating disease and never took the time for myself until the summer of July 2017, when I decided to take flight to Las Vegas, Nevada. It took eight whole years for me to realize that I deserve to explore the world; to live, and it was such an amazing trip and I was able to unwind for four nights and five days without any distractions. This brought a delightful feeling back to my life and I enjoyed every moment. While away I took time to learn how to relax without the phone calls, text or emails of helping others cope with their illnesses.

Every women should find ways to live, laugh, and love again because there's still life after cancer. Sometimes it's just a matter of attending support groups with other women whom have/had breast cancer to be reassured. Many times group sessions can help build one's confidence to comprehend the knowledge and collaborate with other people whom have been through similar illnesses. Being able to live in the moment, love beyond words, and have everlasting laughter everyday certainly helps to fight to survive and have a meaningful life afterwards.

As an 8-year breast cancer survivor, it feels great to attend events and celebrate such victories of survival with other breast cancer survivors as a great milestone to polish up the beginning of a new life pathway. I enjoy encouraging women to stop being afraid of what could go wrong and to focus more on what could go right! Life is like a camera, and women should focus on what's important, remember to capture all the good times life has to offer, spend time with positive people, and if things don't work out just strive at other endeavors to make life worth living. Once in a while, right in the middle of the ordinary life, love offers us a fairy tale. Sometimes it feels good to live like there is no tomorrow because everyone deserves to be happy. Being able to fight for your life and having a personal testimony of a battle with breast cancer and going through the healing process helps to promise yourself to live life to the fullest, love truthfully and laughter will make the greatest difference to feel so much better. I once was so angry and afraid of life or the lack thereof, but it took cancer to help me realize what an amazing, yet strong person I have become in this journey. I never understood the meaning of the word strength until I had no choice but to fight for my life. This cancer journey has made me strong, but I am confident that I would not have made it through without such an amazing support of family and friends.

Being able to live, laugh, learn, and love after breast cancer could be hard at times. Some days trying to readjust and deal with all the fear and anxiety could be stressful, but knowing how to simply relax and breathe again is so joyful and it feels so good inside. Life after cancer isn't an easy road to recovery because there are so many physical scars on my body to remind me of all which I had to go through during the recovery process, but I survived! I was able to survive because of all of the other women whom I inspire each and every day. To hear such sweet words like, "You inspire me so much" and a simple, "thank you" does something to my spirit. Such statements make me realize that my survivorship has enlighten others and my living is not in vain.

Listed below are some ideas to rethink on how to live life well after breast cancer:

- **Unite with women in your community to stand up strong**
- **Enhance your quality of life**
- **Share your experience of healing process**
- **Live a peaceful free lifestyle**

- **Share a treatment care kit for someone you love**

- **Take time for you (travel, pamper yourself)**

There is so much which I can pour into the lives of others fighting the battle against cancer but having a life after cancer is a lifesaving reason to embrace others with my profound love so they will let go of the memories of such an uncomfortable situation.

Chapter 7

Spirituality: A Period of Longsuffering

Romans 5:3-4

"More that, we rejoice in our sufferings, knowing that suffering produces endurance, and endurance produces character, and character produces hope." Longsuffering, or patience, the fourth fruit of the Spirit, it is someone who had to endure something unpleasant, one who had to endure with a long illness but who did it so cheerfully. In many cases, long sufferings is just the test of your faith.

Matthew 17:20

"And Jesus said unto them, Because of your unbelief: for verily I say unto you, "If ye have faith as a grain of mustard seed, ye shall say unto this mountain, Remove hence to yonder place; and it shall remove; and nothing shall be impossible unto you." It is proven to strengthen your faith, so therefore one has to keep on rejoicing even through their long suffering. Once you are united and connected with the Lord and Savior, keep on rejoicing no matter of the hardships which you are going through because your sufferings are not your own but the sufferings of Christ.

Matthew 27:32-56

Imagine the crucifixion of Jesus, when they hung him on the cross and all the pain & anguish he must have felt prior to & during his crucifixion. The longsuffering Jesus probably felt had to be extremely painful. The spirit of glory and of God resting on you is a means of longsuffering which may allow you to think you may not be able to bare it, but if you are a believer of Christ, you will be able to bare all or any illness, in the name of Jesus!

1 Corinthians 10:13

"There hath no temptation taken you, but such as is common to man: but God is faithful, who will not suffer you to be tempted above that you are able: but will with the temptation also make a way to escape, that ye may be able to bear it." In other words, God won't put any more on you than you can bare! Glorifying God helps one to keep rejoicing in suffering because giving God the praise glorifies God and it shows by your actions and attitudes that God is glorious to you, that he is valuable, he's precious, he's desirable, and He's a satisfying God. God's faithfulness to care for our souls is part of the healing process and his healing power to help us all get through the longsuffering. In the midst of all your long sufferings, you will be able to take back & bounce back from all that the enemy has stolen from you.

Joel 2:25

"And I will restore to you the years that the locust hath eaten, the cankerworm, and the caterpillar, and the palmerworm, my great army which I sent among you." Therefore, don't allow the enemy to keep you bound.

Isaiah 54:17

"No weapon that is formed against thee shall prosper; and every tongue that shall rise against thee in judgment thou shalt condemn. This is the heritage of the servants of the Lord, and their righteousness is of me, saith the Lord."

At one point of my life I began to grow to love butterflies without knowing the real true meaning. Butterflies represent a process of hope, vibrant joy, change and a new transformation of healing. I had to spend time in my cocoon and allow God to nurture me through a healing process. I was a woman whom had to pull herself together but once was in a dark place. In spite of that, I realized that there was still hope. I realized that God was preparing me because four years later in 2013 my mother was diagnosed with cancer and I was able to help her cope with her illness. Then, five years after that in 2014, my father transition and my sister-in-law was diagnosed in 2015 with breast cancer. But today even after eight years later, I am a living testimony! I am more than a conqueror. I am healthy & still standing and no more longsuffering!

Hebrews 11:1

"Now faith is the substance of things hoped for, the evidence of things not seen. Hope is the state which promotes the desire of positive outcomes related to certain circumstances or illnesses in one's life." Hope is helping other people embrace. Why? Because embracing someone or supporting someone helps them get through their battle.

Now hope is a powerful thing! Without HOPE you lose your joy, without HOPE you lose your peace of mind, without HOPE you lose confidence but through it all there's still HOPE at the end of the tunnel. The overall outcome is based on the reasons to fight to live and not die. Our confidence in the Lord provides hope. Our commitment to the Lord provides Hope. Living our lives faithfully to the Lord provides a measure of hope that could otherwise never exist.

Our comfort in the Lord provides Hope. We need to realize that the battle is not ours, give it to God and He will help us overcome our struggles, battles and/or illness of infirmity and disease.

Spirituality and prayer is much needed for women especially when going through breast cancer. Sometimes women begin to feel unwanted or unattractive during their life changing experience. It impacts the lives of women's spiritual wellbeing and trying to readjust their look, peace of mind and faith. This puts women of greatness in a time of hardship and it makes their transition feel like their whole world has been put on hold. I've met so many women who have survived breast cancer and looks at me as a women of empowerment to help them cope through such a dreadful, yet devastating time in their lives. This is a disease whom one bravely faces with extraordinary courage! It takes many countless hours of hope, prayer, spirituality or faith in a greater powerful profound love to connect closer to God. One's spirituality makes a big difference in the lives of many women in coping with their illness; how their illness changed their lives tremendously but their spiritual faith can help patients recuperate from breast cancer. Women's use of spirituality helps manifest their prayer life and receive a better connection with God to help guide them through their illness and gain support from others in their own faithful community areas.

Spirituality is a much strongly needed factor in one's life to be able to cope with their illness from diagnosis through treatment, survival, recurrence, and death. During the healing process, it causes stress for some women and it could trigger a deep profound suffering and distress. I look at the women who have been affected by breast cancer and I feel very proud of them because after so many battles faced some lost and others defeated, I believe they are strong warriors with a willingness to fight. Women of strength should be able to stand and have great faith and allow no one or nothing to bring them down because God is the one who sustains all warriors.

Having a means of spiritualty determines how it will make a difference in the lives of women trying to adjust when receiving the dreadful news, "YOU HAVE CANCER!" I had cancer, it was a terrible and a devastating illness. I suffered fatigue and weakness. I lost most of my physical strength. There was fear in the eyes of my family. There were many dark days of agony but my body resisted, endured, and my mental strength lingered and fear subsided. There were more people praying for me than myself! I knew God loved me and with Him by my side, there was nothing that couldn't be beat. But this journey of healing really strengthened my walk with Christ. At this point in my life, I know how to live on almost nothing or with everything! I have learned the secret of living in every situation, whether it is with a full stomach or empty, with plenty or little. I believe in Philippians 3: 12-13 which states, "For I can do everything with the help of Christ who gives me the strength I need." Those that experience the infirmity disease of different types of cancers need spiritual guidance in order to have a continuous mindset to believe the word God.

Isiah 53:1

Who hath believed our report? And to whom is the arm of the lord revealed? I believe the report of the Lord and "SHONDO", God turn my health around and I'm Cancer-Free and won the Victory.

Proverbs 3:8

This will bring health to your body and nourishment to your bones. Every woman should partner up with at least one other woman to talk about their longsuffering journal, emotions and lower level of depressions. I think when a woman can discuss their illness with someone that's trustworthy, it helps ease their mindsets concerning side effects, treatment options, reconstruction and every risk factor to give them hope. Sometimes survivors must ask themselves "Can these Dry Bones Live"?

Ezekiel 37: 1-7

"The hand of the LORD was upon me, and carried me out in the spirit of the LORD, and set me down in the midst of the valley which was full of bones, and caused me to pass by them round about: and, behold, there were very many in the open valley; and, lo, they were very dry. And he said unto me, Son of man, can these bones live? And I answered, O Lord GOD, thou knowest. Again he said unto me, Prophesy upon these bones, and say unto them, O ye dry bones, hear the word of the LORD. Thus saith the Lord GOD unto these bones; Behold, I will cause breath to enter into you, and ye shall live: And I will lay sinews upon you, and will bring up flesh upon you, and cover you with skin, and put breathe in you, and ye shall live; and ye shall know that I am the LORD." When you look around and your illness seems hopeless, often times that's where we go wrong, so where is your faith? When was the last time you activated your faith? When everything in life seems too go wrong, it is then when we should activate and hold on to our faith!

Matthew 27th Chapter

When Jesus was nailed to the cross and all the pain & anguish he must have felt prior to and during his crucifixion had to be horrifying. Our God bared His life on the cross for us and He had to go through and suffer for our sins. Our lives can sometimes be placed in a sham as unexpected tragedy often occurs. We may see ourselves in a valley of dead, dry bones. When you look at your situation and all you see is a valley of dead, dry bones, it's hard to have much hope! It's hard to imagine those dead, dry bones having life. It's hard to imagine your situation ever getting better. It's hard to imagine life beyond our present circumstances. "Can these bones live?" I can truly say I don't look like what I've been through but

God allowed these bones to live. So whose report will you believe?

I believe the report of the Lord and it's because of what He brought me through! If God wants these dead, dry bones to live, they'll live! I receive referrals all the time to talk to other cancer patients about what to expect throughout their treatments. But I'm not a certified counselor, I have no degree or certifications in this field, but through my personal experience of receiving a cancer diagnosis and enduring a painful, gruesome healing experience, I can certainly clarify that healing is possible and through faith, one's hope can be restored!

Chapter 8

Winning the Battle

Winning the battle against breast cancer is a great feeling! In fact, there's no greater feeling of overcoming an obstacle that statistically could have or should have killed me! There's nothing impossible because with much prayer, love and courage anyone can and will win the battle over cancer! I had to fight hard to win the battle of cancer as it took every ounce of strength. I shed so many tears day and night until I was gasping for air but I managed to bounce back even tougher. It was a very difficult time in my life but somehow I managed to regain strength and every year I try to celebrate. I believe I am a strong woman because part of winning the battle against cancer is hope, faith, determination, strength and to keep striving to be great. Having the power to fight, win and overcome is why I am able to be a conqueror and never look back on the journey because I am a strong faith fighter and survivor! It is known that even warriors must face battles. These tough battles such as cancer will cause depression, stressfulness, anxiety, fatigue and there are times you just want to give up but I had to push myself so I could someday say, "I won the fight back against Cancer." So here I am today, celebrating life as an eight (8) year Stage II Beast Cancer Survivor and so energetic and eager to help others cope with their illnesses. I would not have ever thought that such a disease could have invaded and crept into my body but I soon realized that I am one tough chic because I managed to walk away. There are so many journals in life that we all have to face but I don't ever want to face cancer ever again. I can truly say, "Lord I Thank You for my Life".

There were days that I felt like giving up but I kept striving and praying because I knew by His stripes I would be healed. Winning the battle of cancer is not easy but I was determined to live and not die.

To all survivors and other cancer patients know that there are brighter days ahead and you truly deserve to have a healthy life but you must use every ounce of energy to become cancer-free.

To all CAREGIVERS, please know that we are so appreciative for all you do and all the countless hours, support and love to help us along the way. I know for sure I am so thankful for the many friends and family members who were my greatest supporters and still today will be there for me 100% anytime I need them for support. As I think back over my life and all that I had to go through, I truly can say today that I don't look like what I've been through! I made a decision to live and fight and I'm so thankful to God for allowing me to connect, embrace and inspire so many great people. It was my own personal experience and illness that has helped me to gain strength, courage, and confidence to face all my fears. I'm blessed to live a productive life and live life to the fullest, no matter what happens. For I am faithful to God and "Jesus" will take real good care of me. It is well! It feels good to have a spiritual rebirth, vibrant joy, and a new transformation period in life. It's very difficult to say whether we're winning the battle against breast cancer but sometimes you find a new way to win the war.

Chapter 9

A Survivor's Journey of Hope

God began to pour into me on this journey more and more each day. I am grateful to be a survivor of the dreadful disease. Each year on July 23rd, I have a celebration for one more milestone of hope. It's never anything formal or fancy but just to be with a few family members and friends. It's so amazing and it really brightens my day but you only live once so why not show Satan he was defeated? It was a story of triumph, courage and the will to not only survive but thrive. As I think back to the day in December 2015, when I thought my life was starting to get back on the right track, out of nowhere, I had to face another battle and had no clue of the outcome. A modern woman that has both feet on the ground, trying to walk in faith, I had to ask myself, "Whose report will you believe"? Well, on this day, I received a phone call but I continue to pray and kept smiling because I believe the report of the Lord!

Even warriors must face many battles but why fight along when God can fight your battle. The infirmity disease "cancer" that the devil tried to invade in my body had no power to break me because I was covered by the blood of Jesus. I began to go to the doctor for seven (7) long months, taking test after test from December 2015-July 2016. At this moment, my physicians saw low to moderate signs of cancer. I was completely shocked! I couldn't believe that I was possibly going to go through the cancer process again! This moment of crisis in my life was getting me burdened down so therefore I knew I had to reach out to some strong prayer warriors. After being overwhelmed for so many months, I received the news on July 29, 2016 and there were no more signs of cancer. It was like a ton of bricks lifted and I was able to stand again! I did not know how in the world I was going to be able to fight another episode of cancer without being bitter, saddened and fighting not for myself but for others. My passion for helping others is real and I genuinely love helping people in the community. So, to hear that I was once again cancer free was relieving! Through it all, one thing I know for sure is that I never lost my praise. I never lost my hope. I never lost my joy. I never lost my focus. And most of all, I never lost my faith nor did I ever lose my praise!

Inspirational Messages of Hope

During this journey of survival, I began to meditate with God on how my life journey has inspired so many people and it was because of my family and friends that kept me lifted up. I immediately reached out to some of them and ask them to send me inspirational quotes, "As a Caregiver" or "As a Survivor" to let others know just how much they will need a good support system to fight through the battle of cancer. It is because of my family and friends that are so dear to me that I was able to "Win the Fight" and become cancer free for victory! I am victorious and love being a breast cancer mentor to so many who needs help to go through the process. Helping others through the fight to be strong, often times is not an easy task because some of the patients transition and I was so saddened but I know I made a difference in their lives along the way.

I'm so grateful for my team of warriors that backed me up from day one. As a survivor, helping families cope is not an easy task. Sometimes the best way to survive is to share our faith, trust, and simply share our lives and stories. Being a cancer free survivor is not about me but what I can do to help others cope and try to balance the feelings of pain to move forward with their daily lives. I'm thankful because God allowed me to live because of the great works the Lord has on my life. Often times when a patient tries to have a good spirit and allows me to clarify, pray and discuss any concerns of their health issues, it makes room for them to lift the burdens and grow spiritually.

Inspirational Quotes
By
Caregivers & Survivors

As I look upon you as you endure this journey you are showing me just how strong you are. Even though your body is being attacked you're still smiling through the pain. You are reminding me that while you're going through you are not giving up. "You continue to trust God through the storm because you know who calms the storm."

~April O'Neil/As A Caregiver ~

"I will give out before I give up."

~Miranda Brown/As A Survivor ~

"Through prayer, faith and hope all things are Possible!" *~Dr. Nicky E. Collins/As A Survivor ~*

"Accept the things you cannot change, change the things you can, and ask God for strength, peace, and victory through the process."

~Juan Cox/As A Caregiver ~

"Your strength remains unknown until you get up and fight with faith, courage and prayer."

~Antarious D. Wilson/As A Caregiver ~

"Give a smile, a hug and be a great listener. Even though the journey maybe a little rough, let's keep traveling together, making memories, sharing laughs and hugs. And remember to always make time to do things that make "them smile" or "make them happy". *~Anonymous/As A Caregiver ~*

Nothing is impossible with God.

~Marsha Hines/As A Survivor ~

Jeremiah 29:11 assures us that God has positive plans for each of us. Focus on the beauty and the message hidden in your experience. Remember when you look good, you feel good! "Always let your light shine bright, because someone is out there searching for a sign." *~Donna Gibson/As A Caregiver ~*

"Your deliverance can still take place, just have faith.Appreciate life, love the person you are supporting because every scar is just a friendly reminder that I survived."

~Laticia Renee Shaw-Hall/As A Survivor~

"The Lord is the one who writes our story, he can Erase cancer from the life of a cancer victim. We know that the victory has already been won so trust the one who has the Pen in his hand, it's who writes every one of our stories. Sometime your story will include some pain and some sickness but my God is able if you know him like Mary and Martha knew him, but did not trust him. I pray that today you will put all of your trust in him because just as he brought Lazarus back, he can bring you back. Trust him with all your heart and lean not to your own understanding for God is able if you only believe. ~ *Anonymous*

From the desk of a Pastor/As a Caregiver ~

"Cherish the good days, because there will be good days and those are memories you will take with you and survive. "

~Miranda Lewis/As A Caregiver~

"Keep pushing until you see tomorrow."

~ Kira Brown/As A Caregiver ~

"Courage doesn't always ROAR. Sometimes Courage is that quiet voice at the end of the day saying "I will try again tomorrow."

~ Alondrea Williams/As A Caregiver ~

"Your destiny is greater than your storm."

~Tiffani Dawkins/As A Caregiver ~

"Having faith the size of a mustard seed and speak to the mountain in your life and it shall be removed. Just like the woman with the issue of blood, she had faith, she touched the hem of Jesus garment and was made whole. The word of God says: by Jesus's stripes we are healed, we just have to apply these things to our life and God will see us through."

~ Minister Otis Perkins/As A Caregiver ~

"I believe that a caregiver should spend majority of their energy encouraging the patient, reminding them that this sickness is not unto death and God is in charge of their life and he won't put no more on them than they can bare. We must always remember what he did for Hezekiah, he'll do it for us. We should also be reminded that there are no birds in the air that has a backpack but God feed them every day. **~Evangelist Patricia** *Williams/As A Caregiver~*

"Live life! Don't allow Life to live you!"

~ *Pastor Tyrone Smith/As A Caregiver* ~

"I made a decision to fight and never live in fear! Winning the Battle through Hope, Courage & Strength but giving up was never an option!"

~Shanda L. Wright/As A Survivor~

The Guts, the Glory

On January 10, 2010 I finished my last chemo treatment. This was the most terrifying moment in my life. I remember getting ready for church and not feeling my best but was determined to keep the faith, worship and praise God while trying to endure through the process. After taking a long hot shower and taking a moment to breathe while praying that all would be well. Losing my hair was something I had to except because the chemo meds was so strong but it was one of the side effects. As I think back on this day after my first chemotherapy treatment, I started combing my hair and suddenly notice patches of hair was falling on the floor and I couldn't stop crying. I called my little sister and she immediately came to comfort me. Without her support I would have lost my mind. After arriving in the house of God, a dear friend, and hairstylist notice my hair and offered to give me a free haircut. I was forever so grateful of her kindness. For many days and weeks, I wore a scarf or a wig until I decided it was making me feel so uncomfortable. I could barely smile. So many photos that I had taken were filled with little smirks, but on the inside, I had felt so empty inside. However, because of God's grace and mercy, I survived and my hair grew back like new born baby hair.

Never in my wildest dreams would I have ever Thought of facing cancer. It took months before my strength was renewed and my hair grew back but I cried so many nights. I remember screaming from the top of my lungs because I wanted to give up. I even told my mother that I was not going back for any more treatments because I couldn't tolerate all the side effects and felt like my life was ruin but God.

An Organ Donor

Register at www.dmv.org or www.DonateLifeAZ.org

Going through such an illness crisis, I decided to register and become an organ donor.

I pray I will live a long time but after which I ever transition I want to donate my organs to help save a life or lives.

One (1) organ donor can save eight (8) lives.

- Lungs: Transplanted lungs provide people suffering from diseases like cystic, fibrosis, emphysema and pulmonary embolism with new life and a chance to breathe deeply again.

- Liver: A liver transplant can save the life of someone diagnosed with liver failure, chronic hepatitis, biliary atresia and many other conditions.

- Intestines: An intestinal transplant can save the life of an infant or child affected by congenital conditions like short-gut syndrome.

- Heart: A new heart gives a second chance at life to those affected by conditions like cardiomyopathy, myocarditis and heart disease.

- Kidneys: Transplanted kidneys offer healing to those suffering from diseases like end-stage renal failure and diabetes. A kidney transplant can free someone from the necessity of dialysis.

- Pancreas: A transplanted pancreas can heal a person suffering from diabetes. The pancreas is often transplanted with a kidney because diabetes affects both organs.

A Story of Strength

The Story of Mother-Daughter

Survivors Sylvia Wright

And Shanda Wright

By Sharon Richardson

Watching others fighting the battle of cancer is devastating, extremely devastating if that person is your family member. Sylvia & Shanda who is genuine, humble and one of the most loving persons. So for a person such as themselves to have to go through this sort of test definitely doesn't eliminate the rest of us from far worst. In support of other survivors, the Wright Family found themselves attending and supporting activities whose focus were a cure for cancer. It was in 2009 when Shanda Wright was diagnosed with Stage II Breast Cancer. She endured unilateral mastectomy, chemotherapy treatments, radiation treatments and reconstructive surgeries she soon found herself walking at the Relay for Life & Making Strides for Breast Cancer in her own breast cancer shirt.

A Vision of Sisterhood

Based on her experiences, Shanda had a vision that would bring people together to fight for a cure for cancer, from this The Pink Sistas Organization was born. Right before Shanda's very eyes the Pink Sistas grew in numbers and many doors were opened allowing her the opportunities to tell her story and to Minister to people in all walks of life. Shanda's mother, Sylvia Wright, was there from the very beginning; praying, encouraging, supporting, fundraising, volunteering and helping to form The Pink Sistas. Sylvia did this out of love for her daughter and in hopes that one day it will prevent this from happening to someone else. She also realized this could have happened to her. And it did.

Like Daughter, Like Mother

Sylvia was diagnosed with Stage II Breast Cancer four years later and it could not have come at a more dreadful time in her life. It was during this time Sylvia was the caregiver for her very ill husband, Shanda's father. Because Sylvia watched her daughter will to live and her determination to help others live, she was able to grasp hold to that same concept. They share like experiences, strong determination and work diligently encouraging everyone to get tested regularly, they witness often to cancer victims that there is life after cancer and they do all in their power to seek for a cure!

Moving Forward

Shanda is an eight (8) year survivor, and the Pink Sistas Organization is now called, "The Pink Sistas and Brothers Ministry". She is currently in her fifth year as the Event Chair for the American Cancer Society/Relay for Life of Gadsden County. Sylvia is approaching her fourth year as a survivor; she is an active member of The Pink Sistas and Brothers Ministry and a firm supporter of the Relay for Life. It is their belief that God has a reason for allowing things to happen; we may never understand His wisdom, but we simply have to TRUST HIS WILL for our lives!

Join the Movement

You may not have breast cancer but you still have the power to fight it!

- **Schedule your yearly mammogram**

Women's Imaging Center at Radiology Associates

1600 Phillips Road

Tallahassee, Florida 32308

- **Join in the fight back against Breast Cancer**

Make a Donation:

American Cancer Society

2619 Centennial Blvd #101

Tallahassee, Florida 32308

- **Get involved, participate in Annual Events**

Relay for Life

Sheriff A. Morris Young

Breast Cancer Awareness 35 mile Walk

Making Strides against Breast Cancer

- ***Support***

  Wear Pink in October, Breast Cancer

  Awareness Month

  (In honor of a fallen breast cancer survivor)

Resources

Capital Medical Society, Foundation

"We Care Network"

1204 Miccosukee Road

Tallahassee, Florida 32306

(850) 942-5215

Depending on your medical need, this facility will help pay for medical expensive (surgery and/or medicines) if you do not have any medical insurance upon requested assistance.

Disability Advocates of North Florida

Ms. Leanna Littles

1018 Thomasville Road

Suite # 103-C

Tallahassee, Florida 32303

(850) 893-7970

Most cancer patients can't work while trying to endure the process of treatments. This is a reliable source that will help you file all necessary paperwork to get benefits.

More detailed information will be given at appointment discussion with representative.

TMH "A Woman's Place"

1301 East Sixth Avenue

Tallahassee, Florida 32303

(850) 431-4928

Ask surgical physician if you qualify to get breast prosthesis and bras. This facility offers caring services & quality products designed to support patients. Ask physician for more detailed information.

A National call center

1-800-227-2345 & representatives are willing and available to answer your questions.

The Hope Lodge

It's for people who need a free place to stay while

traveling for treatment, so patients can

save millions of dollars in lodging costs.

Road to Recovery

For people that need a ride to and from their

treatment which volunteers help provide rides for

cancer patients.

Support System

Patients need referrals because after a person has just

heard the dreaded words "You have

Cancer" & need someone to talk too immediately to

who has been there before. Many times women

battling breast cancer are taking life

saving chemotherapy drugs, numerous

treatments of radiation and a four stage step of

reconstruction.

Recommended Physicians

These following physicians are highly recommended that will give good caring services to cancer patients but there are other physicians that have the willingness to provide services and answer any questions necessary.

TMH Southeastern Surgical Group

Dr. Richard Zorn, MD

1401 Centerville Road #100

Tallahassee, Florida 32308

(850) 877-5183

Tallahassee Memorial Cancer Center

Dr. Phillip Sharp/Radiation Oncology

1775 One Healing Place

Tallahassee, Florida 32308, (850) 431-5255

Tallahassee Memorial Cancer Center

Dr. Karen Russell, M.D.-Hematology/Oncology,

Internal Medicine

1775 One Healing Place

Tallahassee, Florida 32308

(850) 431-5360

Southeastern Plastic Surgery, P.A. Cosmetic &

Reconstruction Surgery

Dr. Ben Kirbo, M.D.

2030 Fleischmann Road,

Tallahassee, Florida 32308

(850) 219-2000

Dr. Laurence Z. Rosenberg, M.D.

2030 Fleischmann Road

Tallahassee, Florida 32308

(850) 219-2000

Acknowledgements

This new chapter in my life has been a powerful journey of hope. As stated in previous chapters, I would not have been able to successfully heal without the love and support of family and friends. I would like to personally thank my caregivers Sylvia Wright (mother) and Tiffani Dawkins (sister), for their tireless efforts in caring for me. I would also like to thank my God-Sister Sharon Richardson, sister-in-law Miranda Brown and nephew Antarious Wilson for helping me during visitations and many others. There were a host of prayer warriors fighting on my behalf. Therefore, I would like to thank all family, friends, and pastors for praying for me on my behalf. A special thank you to my dearest friend Raven Rushton for taking the time out of her busy schedule to proofread, edit, and help me get the book publish. I am very thankful to my family and friends that pushed me to believe in myself, knowing that this book will inspire others, give them strength, courage, and much hope to fight. I hope this book inspires other women & men to know that there is still life after cancer.

It is through this book that I pray that I am able to encourage others to keep pushing, pray without ceasing and to NEVER give up hope!

About The Author

Shanda Wright, the woman whom wears many hats is a woman of God, devoted daughter, sister, aunt and a breast cancer survivor. Shanda graduated from James A. Shanks High School in 1986. Then attended Branell Institute in 1991, where she became certified as a Hi-Tech Secretary. She is currently employed as a Paraprofessional at Stewart Street Elementary School in the Gadsden County School District since 2010. Shanda recently decided to further her education as a dual college major in Elementary Education & Special Education; starting in December 2013 and presently attending online college classes at Grand Canyon University, a university that is in alignment with her educational goals and Christian faith. Shanda wants to be able to work with children with special needs & help train them for events such as the Special Olympics.

In 2009, Shanda was diagnosed with stage II breast cancer, but is now an 8 year cancer survivor! The journey of having cancer was a life changing experience that she will never forget. God had definitely spared her life and she believes that it is because her work on earth was not completed. Since enduring this life changing experience, Shanda has chosen to educate others about cancer has become a Motivational Speaker through an organizational group called the Pink Sistas & Brothers Ministry. As the founder of the group, she and her team of volunteers encourage and inspire other women & men to live healthy active lives. In 2015, Shanda also started an additional inspiring challenge "Survivors Look Good, Feel Better Glamour Portraits" to give survivors a makeover and photo-shoot so they will have the opportunity to know that it's not about their outer beauty but there inner beauty to make them feel glamorous.

In her spare time, Shanda loves volunteering with local agencies in the community. She currently held the position as the Event Coordinator for the Annual Sheriff Morris A. Young Breast Cancer Awareness 35 mile Walk in 2016. She was the Online Chair for the Relay for Life of Gadsden in 2012. Now, she currently holds a volunteer leadership position as the Event Lead Chair Person since 2013 for the Relay for Life of Gadsden with American Cancer Society. Shanda also enjoys exercising (walking & running), comedy & action movies, and fellowshipping with Christian believers. My favorite book of all is the King James' Edition of the Bible.

As a Breast Cancer Survivor, Shanda has been blessed with many opportunities to be a motivational/inspirational speaker at various Breast Cancer Awareness programs, encouraging others to never ever give up hope and sharing my survivor story.